PowerUp Smoothie Recipes

Cleanse, Energize, Feel Great

Volume 1

Your Free Gift

I wanted to show my appreciation that you support my work, so I've put together a free gift for you.

http://www.letoilepublishing.com/1smoothie

Just visit the link above to download it now.
I know you will love this gift.

Thanks!
Taylor Golden

Table of Contents

Kale Smoothie

- 16 ounces (2 cups) chopped kale
- 2 ounces (2 cups) Greek yogurt
- 1 ½ ounces peanuts (optional)
- 4 ounces milk
- 1/2 frozen banana
- 3 frozen strawberries, or more to taste
- 1/2 ounces maple syrup

Directions

1. Mix kale, yogurt, and peanuts together in a blender until smooth. Include milk, banana, strawberries, and maple syrup and mix until wanted consistency is reached.

Cook's Notes:

- Substitute any kind of juice for the milk. If you decide to substitute juice for the milk, blend juice with kale, yogurt, and peanuts until smooth. If you over-mix with milk, it may get to be excessively thick and solidified fixings get to be foamy.
- You can utilize any kind of yogurt. Substitute nectar for the maple syrup.

Lemon with Berry Smoothie

Ingredients

- 8 ounces blueberry nonfat yogurt
- 12 ounces skim milk
- 8 ounces ice cubes
- 8 ounces fresh blueberries
- 1 ounce fresh strawberries
- 1/6 ounces powdered lemonade mix

Directions

1. Place yogurt, milk, ice shapes, blueberries, strawberries, and lemonade blend in a blender. Beat until smooth and rich.

Mongolian Strawberry with Orange Juice Smoothie

Ingredients

- 8 ounces chopped fresh strawberries
- 8 ounces orange juice
- 10 cubes ice
- 1/2 ounces sugar

Directions

1. In a blender, combine strawberries, squeezed orange, ice cubes and sugar. Mix until smooth. Put into glasses and serve.

Sweet Potato with Banana Smoothie

Ingredients

- 1 large sweet potato
- 1 banana
- 16 ounces soy milk
- 1/24 ounces ground cinnamon

Directions

1. Preheat stove to 350 degrees F (175 degrees C).
2. Bake sweet potato in the preheated stove until delicate and cooked through, around 1 hour. Expel peel from cooked sweet potato and cool in the fridge 8 hours or overnight.
3. Blend sweet potato, banana, soy milk, and cinnamon together in a blender until smooth.

Cook's Note:

- You can likewise microwave the sweet potato for about 10 minutes instead of baking it.
- Peel the cooked sweet potato before or after cooling it.

Lime with Mango Smoothie

Ingredients

- 3 mangoes, peeled, pitted, and cut into 1-inch chunks
- 1 ounce fresh lime juice
- 1 ounce confectioners' sugar
- 1 tray ice cubes

Directions

1. Place the mangoes, lime squeeze, confectioners' sugar, and ice cubes in a blender. Mix until slushy.

Chocolate Milk Banana Smoothie

Ingredients

- 1 banana
- 1/2 ounces chocolate syrup
- 8 ounces milk
- 8 ounces crushed ice

Directions

1. In a blender, combine banana, chocolate syrup, and milk and squashed ice. Mix until smooth. Put into glasses and serve.

Green Smoothie Slime

Ingredients

- 16 ounces spinach
- 16 ounces frozen strawberries
- 1 banana
- 1 ounce honey
- 4 ounces ice

Directions

1. Place the spinach in the cooler until solidified, at least 1 hour.

2. Combine the spinach, strawberries, banana, nectar, and ice in a blender. Mix until smooth. Serve promptly.

Pineapple with Banana Smoothie

Ingredients

- 4 ice cubes
- 1/4 fresh pineapple - peeled, cored and cubed
- 1 large banana, cut into pieces
- 8 ounces pineapple or apple juice

Directions

1. Spot ice cubes, pineapple, banana, and pineapple juice into the bowl of a blender. Puree on high until smooth.

Raspberry with Blackberry Smoothie

Ingredients

- 1 small banana
- 4 ounces blackberries
- 8 ounces fresh raspberries
- 6 ounces vanilla yogurt
- 1/2 ounces honey
- 4 ice cubes

Directions

1. Place banana, blackberries, raspberries, and yogurt, honey, and ice cubes into a blender. Blend until smooth.

Cinnamon with Pear Smoothie

Ingredients

- 2 pears, quartered and cores removed
- 1 banana, cut in pieces
- 8 ounces milk
- 4 ounces vanilla yogurt
- 1/12 ounces ground cinnamon
- 1 pinch ground nutmeg

Directions

1. Place the pears, banana, milk, yogurt, cinnamon, and nutmeg into a blender. Cover, and puree until smooth. Put into glasses to serve.

Mango with Pineapple Smoothie

Ingredients

- 8 ounces vanilla yogurt
- 8 ounces unsweetened pineapple juice
- 1/2 banana, sliced
- 1 mango - peeled, seeded, and chopped
- 4 ounces nonfat milk
- 1 ounce cream of coconut

Directions

1. In a blender, mix the vanilla yogurt, pineapple juice, banana, mango, milk, and cream of coconut until smooth.

Grapefruit Smoothie

Ingredients

- 10 2/3 ounces fresh red grapefruit juice
- 8 large strawberries
- 2 medium bananas, sliced
- 8 ounce strawberry-banana yogurt
- 1 ounce honey
- 8 ounces crushed ice

Directions

1. Place the grapefruit juice, strawberries, bananas, yogurt, honey, and ice into a blender. Cover, and blend until smooth.

Nectarine Smoothie

Ingredients

- 2 large nectarines, hollowed and quartered
- 1 banana, cut into pieces and frozen
- 1 large orange, peeled and quartered
- 8 ounces vanilla yogurt
- 8 ounces orange juice
- 1/2 ounces honey

Directions

1. Place the nectarines, solidified banana pieces, orange, vanilla yogurt, squeezed orange, and nectar into a blender, and mix until smooth.

Frosted Mocha Milk Shake

Ingredients

- 6 ounces milk
- 1/6 ounces vanilla extract
- 1 1/2 ounces granulated sugar
- 1 1/2 ounces mocha flavored instant coffee mix
- 8 ounces crushed ice

Directions

1. In a blender or food processor, combine milk, vanilla, sugar, espresso powder and smashed ice. Mix until smooth. Put into glasses and serve.

Mango Lassi

Ingredients

- 2 mangos - peeled, seeded and diced
- 16 ounces plain yogurt
- 4 ounces white sugar
- 8 ounces ice

Directions

1. In a blender, combine mangos, yogurt, sugar and ice. Mix until smooth. Put into glasses and serve.

Peanut Butter with Banana Smoothie

Ingredients

- 2 bananas, cut into pieces
- 16 ounces milk
- 4 ounces peanut butter
- 1 ounce honey, or to taste
- 16 ounces ice cubes

Directions

1. Place bananas, milk, peanut butter, nectar, and ice cubes in a blender; mix until smooth, around 30 seconds.

Chamomile, peach with ginger smoothie

Ingredients

- 1 chamomile tea bag
- 4 ounces low-fat or soy milk
- 1 peach, skinned, stone removed
- 1/6 ounces grated fresh ginger
- 1/6-1/3 ounces wheat germ (optional)

Directions

1. Place teabag in a container, spread with 2 2/3 ounces boiling water. Cool, remove bag and spot tea in blender with remaining ingredients. Mix until smooth.

Coconut Milky Avocado Smoothie

Ingredients

- 1 Hass avocado, diced
- 4 ounces low-fat vanilla yogurt
- 4 ounces fresh milk
- 2 ounces coconut cream
- 8 ice cubes

Directions

1. Consolidate avocado, yogurt, milk, cream of coconut, and ice cubes in a blender; mix until smooth.

Cook's Notes:

- Please make sure that you use cream of coconut. It is thick like sweetened consolidated milk. Using coconut milk or coconut water will drastically influence the outcome and should not be used. Cream of coconut can be found in your grocery with the mixed drink blends or with the outside sustenances.

- Add more milk if you like your smoothie more slender, more ice if you like it thicker.

Frozen Fruit Smoothie

Ingredients

- 1 frozen banana, peeled and sliced
- 16 ounces frozen strawberries, raspberries, or cherries
- 8 ounces milk
- 4 ounces plain or vanilla yogurt
- 4 ounces freshly squeezed orange juice
- 1 to 1 1/2 ounces honey

Directions

1. Put all the ingredients in a blender and procedure until smooth. Pour into glasses and serve.

Cook's note:

- For non-dairy smoothies, substitute 8 ounces rice milk for the milk and yogurt. Alternately, use soy yogurt or milk instead of dairy.

Green smoothie

Ingredients

- 8 ounces spinach, trimmed, cleaved, firmly pressed
- 8 ounces chopped kale, trimmed, cleaved, hard pressed
- 4 ounces celery, chopped
- 1/12 ounces cinnamon
- 1 green apple, cored, chopped
- 1 pear, cored, chopped
- 2 large bananas, frozen and roughly chopped
- 16 ounces filtered water
- Fresh mint

Directions

1. Put all ingredients in a blender on high speed and mix until smooth. Divide into 2 tall glasses. Top with fresh mint to serve.

Mango with Passion-fruit Smoothie

Ingredients

- 1 large mango, peeled, flesh roughly chopped
- 8 ounces passion-fruit frozen yoghurt
- 4 ounces milk

Directions

1. Place mango, frozen yoghurt and milk in a blender. Blend until smooth and thick. Put into glasses and serve.

Melon with Strawberry Lassi

Ingredients

- 1/4 small pineapple, peeled, chopped
- 1/8 small rock-melon, peeled, chopped
- 4 3/8 ounces strawberries, hulled
- 2 ounces low-fat yoghurt
- 4 ounces Golden Circle Unsweetened Pineapple Juice
- 1/24 ounces ground cardamom
- 16 ounces ice cubes
- Mint sprigs

Directions

1. Combine fruit in a blender. Blend until smooth.
2. Add yoghurt, pineapple juice, cardamom and ice. Blend until creamy and smooth. Pour into glasses. Garnish with mint sprigs and serve.

Smoothie cubes

Ingredients

- Blackberries, strawberries, raspberries, passion fruit, mango, any other fruits you like

Directions

1. Purée a fruit (blackberries, strawberries, raspberries, passion fruit and mango) in a food processor.
2. Freeze in ice cube trays ready to mix up (3 per serving) with a banana, 5 ounces pot plain yogurt, and milk and honey to taste.

Pineapple Green Smoothie

Ingredients

- 4 ounces unsweetened almond milk
- 2 2/3 ounces nonfat plain Greek yogurt
- 8 ounces baby spinach
- 8 ounces frozen banana slices
- 4 ounces frozen pineapple chunks
- 1/2 ounces chia seeds
- 1/6-1/3 ounces pure maple syrup or honey (optional)

Directions

1. Add almond milk and yogurt to a blender, and then add spinach, banana, pineapple, chia and sweetener. Blend until smooth.

Salad Smoothie

Ingredients

- 8 ounces water, or as desired
- 1/2 orange, peeled
- 8 ounces fresh spinach
- 1/2 raw beet, peeled
- 2 2/3 ounces baby carrots
- 2 2/3 ounces cauliflower florets
- 2 2/3 ounces broccoli florets
- 2 ounces blueberries
- 1 stalk celery
- 1/2 lime, peeled
- 1/2 ounces honey
- 1/2 ounces chia seeds

Directions

1. Put water into the pitcher of a high-controlled blender; include the orange, spinach, beet, carrots, cauliflower, broccoli, blueberries, and celery, lime, nectar, and chia seeds. Mix on fast until smooth, around 1 minute.

Your Free Gift

I wanted to show my appreciation that you support my work, so I've put together a free gift for you.

http://www.letoilepublishing.com/1smoothie

Just visit the link above to download it now.
I know you will love this gift.

Thanks!
Taylor Golden